VITAMINS, MINERALS, ENZYMES, FREE RADICALS, ANTIOXIDANTS

By
Dr. Neo

Table of Contents

ABOUT THE BOOK

By pointing out some facts about these minute and seemingly insignificant components of our nutrients known as vitamins and minerals, we become aware of the essential role they play in the proper functioning of our body.

We learn to appreciate and value their contribution to a healthier and happier life. This book was created exactly for this reason.

For more information, please visit:

www.DrNeoHealing.com

FOREWORD

Dr. Neo, a successful holistic medicine practitioner, has come up with his new book *VITAMINS, MINERALS, ENZYMES, FREE RADICALS, ANTIOXIDANTS*.

Although many books and articles have been written about them, Dr. Neos's book offers a more readable treatment of the subject that can be appreciated by health professionals and laymen alike.

VITAMINS, MINERALS, ENZYMES, FREE RADICALS, ANTIOXIDANTS discusses many of the well-known (as well as the little known) facts about these minute but powerful substances that play a big part in the health and well being of people. Dr. Neo is a staunch advocate of bringing health consciousness to a greater number of people so he has written this book in a way that it can be appreciated by those seriously studying vitamins like medical professionals and students and by readers who merely seek additional knowledge about the topic like the housewives and lay health enthusiasts.

This book is based on Dr. Neo's personal knowledge and experiences as a medical practitioner and combined with the latest findings on vitamins by medical experts in the field of nutrition. He explains the seeming complexities of vitamins in clearer terms and debunks old myths about them, thus assuring his readers of updated information on the subject.

With this book, Dr. Neo is able to attain his goal of advocating holistic health care by highlighting the important roles these minute but potent substances play in maintaining a person's well-being.

Dr. Neo dedicates this book to you, his readers, and wishes you all good health now and through the years to come!

INTRODUCTION

This book **"VITAMINS, MINERALS, ENZYMES, FREE RADICALS, ANTIOXIDANTS"** discusses the importance of a group of organic and inorganic substances found in foods that enable the body to work properly. They are known as VITAMINS, organic substances that are derived from plants and animals; and MINERALS, inorganic elements that come from the soil and water which are absorbed by plants or eaten by animals. These vitamins and minerals work synergistically to sustain life, promote growth, and help cells and organs do their jobs. They also boost the immune system.

In addition to these functions, vitamins and minerals help maintain the body's proper functions by acting as antioxidants like the vitamins A, C, E, and the mineral selenium are. As antioxidants, these substances form as the defense system of the body that inhibits the formation of free radicals.

Free radicals are atoms with odd number of electrons which are formed when oxygen interacts with certain molecules. They turn into highly reactive radicals which can start a chain reaction that cause cellular damage such as cancer, aging, and a variety of diseases.

Chapter 1

VITAMINS

Vitamins are known as organic chemical compounds found in small quantities in food which are necessary for an organism to maintain its metabolism, growth and customary function. In 1912 the word vitamin was derived from the word "vitamine" to define the newly discovered class of substances at that time. Initially, vitamins were thought to be all amines which were indispensable to life. Hence, the first part of the word is derived from the word '*vita*' which in Latin means '*life*'. However, it was noted that not all vitamins were amines. This was why the "e" at the end of the word was dropped.

The organic structures of the vitamins are all known so they can all now being synthetically reproduced in laboratories; the manufactured vitamins are structurally the same as their natural counterparts in nutrients. The Recommended Dietary Allowance (RDA) of each vitamin is the standard recommendation presented by the Food and Nutrition Board, National Academy of Sciences–National Research Council. A well-balanced intake of vitamin supplements typically meets the minimum vitamin requirements of humans. This result is based on the dietary requirements of an ordinary person in good health.

Vitamins A, B complex, C, D, E and K fall in the category of either fat-soluble or water-soluble vitamins. The letters absent amongst them and the omitted numbers in vitamin B complex is because there were some substances that were initially assumed to be vitamins but were gradually eliminated from the list by nutritionists for several reasons. One of them was because they were initially assumed to be necessary but subsequent studies concluded that the body was producing them in adequate amounts. This was also the reason why the symbols of vitamins skipped from E to K.

Initially, vitamins were categorized based on their solubility in water or fats, but as more were detected later, vitamins were further grouped alphabetically. A, D, E, and K were discovered to be fat soluble vitamins while the B complex and C vitamins were water soluble. A group of elements that reduces blood vessel fragility known as the P group was discovered but these were not regarded as vitamins anymore.

2.1. FAT-SOLUBLE VITAMINS

Falling under this categories are vitamins A, D, E and K. These fat-soluble vitamins are absorbed within the abdominal tract with the aid of fats (lipids). They are gathered in the liver and adipose tissues. Fat-soluble vitamins are easier to store than water-soluble ones and can remain in the body as reserved minerals for days, or even for some of them, even months. These vitamins that stay in the system for quite a while may pose a higher threat for toxicity when taken in excess. However, a sensible and healthy diet usually helps in ensuring that only the sufficient amount of them is consumed.

Fortunately, intake of inadequate amounts of these compounds is rare but in case it happens, it is usually due to unhealthy diet or medical complications. These may decrease the absorption of fats which consequently diminish the absorption of these vitamins.

2.1.1. VITAMIN A

Chemical names for this vitamin include Retinol or A1 which is required for protein synthesis and 3-dehydroretionol or A2 which prevents night impaired vision; It is also known as beta-carotene which is found in carrots and plants and is transformed into vitamin A in the human body.

The typical requirement of Vitamin A in grown-ups amounts to 700-900 mcg/day. This quantity could increase if hyperthyroidism, cold, anxiety, excess sunbeam exposure, alcohol, and renal deficiency are present. Toxicity can occur if the dose exceeds 3000mcg per day with symptoms such as dry skin, headache, nausea, loss of appetite and vertigo. Expectant women are at risk of developing birth deficiencies and liver toxicity. Deficiency of Vitamin A, on the other hand, may cause night-blindness and keratomalacia (eye dry cornea condition). Moreover, in children this vitamin plays a major role in deficient teeth growth and slower bone development.

Vitamin A sources include liver, cod liver oil, carrot, broccoli, sweet potato, butter, kale, spinach, pumpkin, collard greens, some cheeses, egg, apricot, cantaloupe melon and milk.

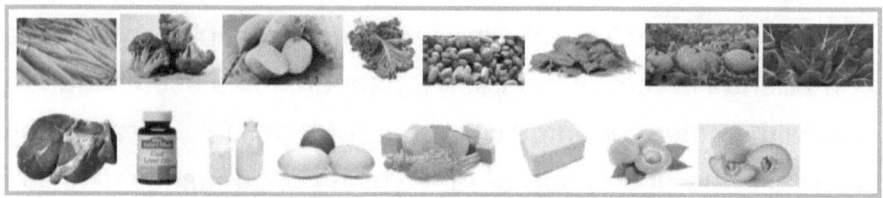

2.1.2. VITAMIN D

Ultraviolent radiation from the sun on an individual's skin aids in the production of Vitamin D in the body. Chemical names for this vitamin are Calciferol (activated Ergosterol), and D2 This radiation increases the absorption of calcium and phosphorus from the small intestine and stimulates 7-dehydrocholesterol. Vitamin D is also known as D3 which prevents rickets (extensive soft bent legs). Overall, vitamin D plays an important role in cell protection and development of the body. It helps children, too, to grow strong bones and teeth.

Sun exposure for 10-15 minutes two times a week is sufficient to meet the body's vitamin D requirement which amounts to 15mcg/day. Other sources of vitamin D are fatty fish, cod liver and beef liver, mushrooms, eggs and dairy products.

Excess intake of more than 150mcg daily, however, can cause liver toxicity, slow development, queasiness, loss of appetite and vomiting. Furthermore, excess amounts of

Vitamin D in adults can also cause osteomalacia (muscle and bone weakness) and osteoporosis (less bone mass), as well as cancer, autoimmune diseases and contagions. In children, excess of the vitamin may result to rickets and flattening of the back of the skull. In northern countries, people are more likely to develop vitamin D deficiency because of the scarcity of sunlight.

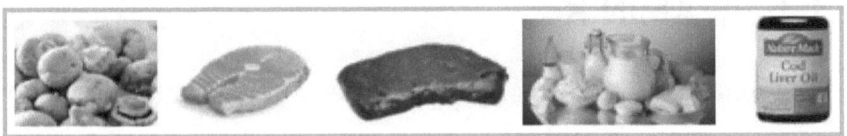

2.1.3. VITAMIN E

Vitamin E is also referred to as tocopherols and tocotrienols. It is considered a superior antioxidant and it safeguards vitamins A and C, as well as the red blood cells. It also protects vital fatty acids from mutilation.

The recommended daily requirement for Vitamin E in adults is about 15 mcg. Excess in use is not harmful, unless there is specific drug interaction with courmadin and other static drugs. Even though Vitamin E deficiency is rare, it can arise in premature new-borns, people with health complications who are unable to absorb fat, or because of unhealthy diets due to reduced fats in them.

Sources of this vitamin are corn, cottonseed and safflower, dairy products, eggs, fruits, vegetables, vegetable oils such as soybean, nuts like almond hazelnuts, seeds, and fortified cereals.

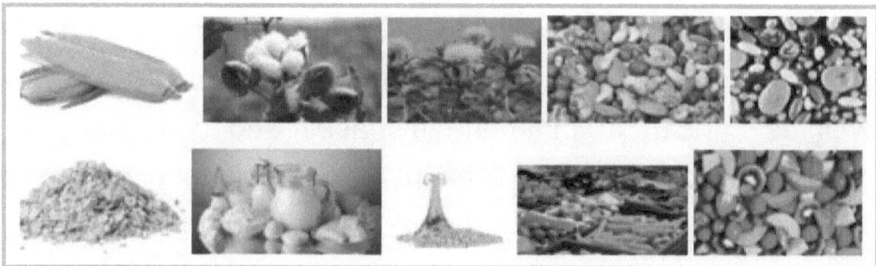

2.1.4. VITAMIN K

This vitamin, also known as phylloquinone and menaquinones, is naturally produced by the bacteria in the intestines. It is an important factor for the process of normal blood clotting. It also aids in the production of protein for blood, kidneys and bones. Breakdown of red blood cells and liver are possible negative effects if the intake of vitamin K is taken in excess. On the other hand, insufficient dose of it may cause deficiency in infants and adults taking medical drugs such as anticoagulants and antibiotics.

Natural sources of vitamin K are vegetables such as spinach, broccoli, cauliflower, cabbage and, specifically, parsley. Even though animal food contains minimal amounts of this vitamin, other sources include fruit, olive, soybean, cottonseed and vegetable oils such as canola.

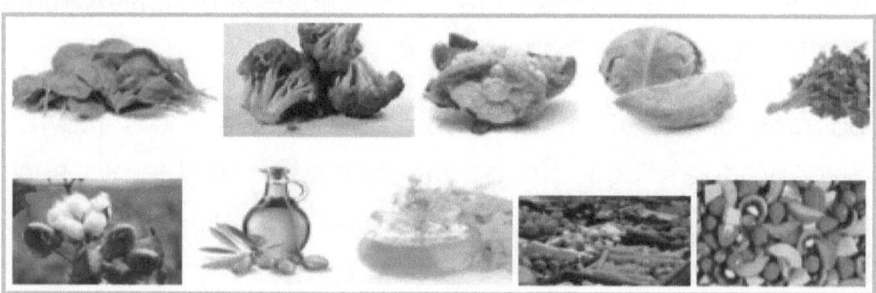

2.2. WATER-SOLUBLE VITAMINS

Under this category fall Vitamins B complex and C. Water-soluble vitamins have short body storage life and can dissolve in water. These vitamins are not stored in the body and are gradually excreted through urine. It is important, therefore, that they are replenished more frequently than the fat-soluble ones. Since any excess in the intake of water-soluble vitamins are excreted by the body with the urine, they do not cause overdose and hence, do not pose any health risk. Water-soluble vitamins are derived from plant and animal foods or can be taken daily as dietary supplements.

2.2.1. VITAMIN B COMPLEX

Vitamins B are a group of water-soluble vitamins that can be obtained from seeds, eggs, vegetables yeast, germs, liver and flesh. They are vital to the metabolic processes of animals, i.e., in the absorption of amino acids and the prevention of skin and nerve disorders. Vitamin B also functions as a shield for diseases such as pernicious anemia (failure of red blood cell production). It also plays a part in nucleic-acid synthesis, fat metabolism, and the transformation of starch to fat. Most of the vitamins in this group are co-enzymes, meaning that they are co-factors with enzymes in stimulating a range of metabolic reactions.

2.2.1.1. VITAMIN B1 (THIAMINE)

Vitamin B1, otherwise known as Thiamine, is crucial for carbohydrate metabolism and aids in the proper function of enzymes. Absence of vitamin B1 may contribute to developing beriberi (a condition involving the heart, nerves, and gastric disorders). Cancer patients who take too much of vitamin B1 can also be at risk of triggering the cancer cells to develop faster.

Sources of this vitamin include brown rice, whole grain rye, asparagus, kale, cauliflower, potatoes, oranges, liver, eggs, pork, cereal grains and sunflower seeds.

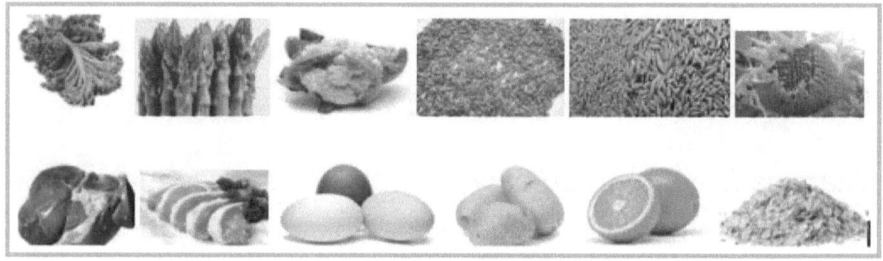

2.2.1.2. VITAMIN B2 (RIBOFLAVIN)

Also known as Riboflavin, vitamin B2 transfers oxygen to the cells. It is also vital for all flavour-proteins which are the proteins absorbed by the elimination of radicals, photosynthesis, DNA restoration, and apoptosis. Moreover, Riboflavin aids in energy absorption and in the metabolism of fats, carbohydrates and proteins. It is also essential for the proper functioning of some enzymes and for maintaining healthy skin, strong nails, and hair. Lack of Riboflavin may result to ariboflavinosis, a disorder that can cause skin, mouth or eye infections.

Good food sources of vitamin B2 are okra, chard, cottage cheese, milk, asparagus, bananas, persimmons, yogurt, meat, eggs, fish, and green beans.

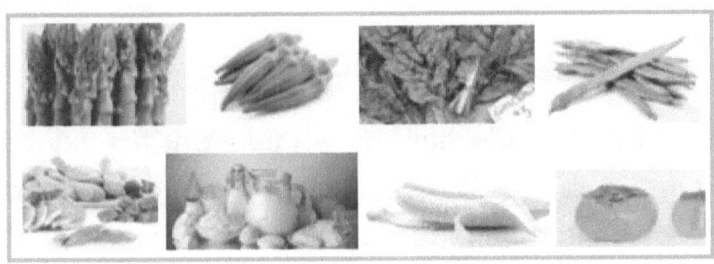

2.2.1.3. VITAMIN B3 (NIACIN)

Other names for vitamin B3 include niacin or nicotinic acid and niacinamide. This vitamin is known to enhance the levels of good cholesterol (HDL) and lower that of triglycerides. Additionally, it fights cancer cells and aids in the proper function of enzymes. Skin, nerves, and the digestive system may benefit from vitamin B3 by keeping them healthy.

Deficiency of this vitamin may cause pellagra, a disorder relating to skin, nerve, and digestive conditions.

Milk, eggs, avocados, dates, tomatoes, leafy vegetables, broccoli, carrots, liver, heart, kidney, chicken, beef, fish (tuna, salmon), sweet potatoes, asparagus, nuts, whole grains, legumes, mushrooms, and brewer's yeast are good sources of vitamin B3.

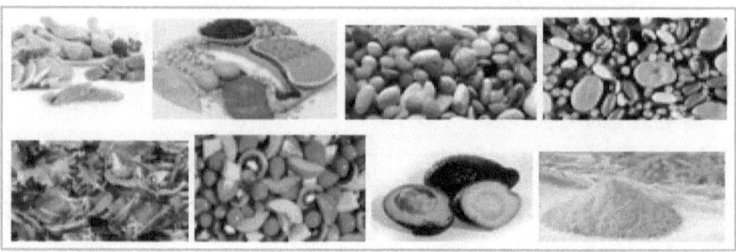

2.2.1.4. VITAMIN B4 (CHOLINE)

Vitamin B4 or Choline has many important functions in the body. One is in the formation of neurotransmitter Acetylo-Choline which is required for muscle development and brain function. Another is its part in the formation of Phosphati-Dylo-Choline which is indispensable for cell tissue integrity. Choline is involved in the creation of Sphingomyelin. This is crucial for the shielding and proper operation of the nervous system. Vitamin B4 regulates liver function and reduces inessential fat residues due to its lipotrophic properties.

Some of the conditions attributed to the deficiency of vitamin B4 are Alzheimer which is a memory issue, Parkinsons, Cardiovascular Diseases, Anxiety, Attention Deficit Hyperactivity Disorder (ADHD), Hypertension, Schizophrenia, Alcoholism, Cirrhosis, Multiple Sclerosis, Amyotrophic Lateral Sclerosis (ALS), Arthrosclerosis, Epilepsy, high level of bad Cholesterol (LDL), HyperTricyglerydemia, infertility, and birth deficiencies.

Sources of Vitamin B4 include shrimp, eggs, scallops, chicken, turkey, cod, tuna, salmon, beef and collard greens.

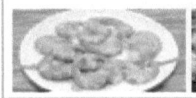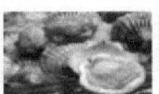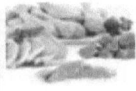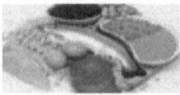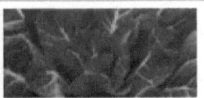

2.2.1.5. VITAMIN B5 (PANTOTHENIC ACID)

Vitamin B5, known also as Pantothenic Acid, supports the breakdown of fats and starches to glucose. It is very important for the production of cholesterol and the development of red blood cells. Lack of vitamin B5 can result to nausea, exhaustion, sleeplessness, melancholy, and tetchiness, stomach aches, burning feet, and upper respiratory infections.

Good food sources of vitamin B5 are shiitake mushrooms (which contain 50% of Vitamin B5), avocado, sweet potato, lentils, chicken, broccoli, and yogurt.

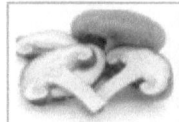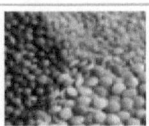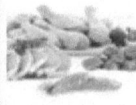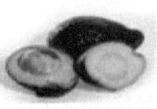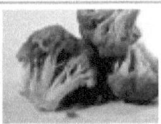

2.2.1.6. VITAMIN B6 (PYRIDOXINE)

The decarboxylation of amino acids requires Pyridoxin, known as Vitamin B6. Pyridoxine aids in the production of certain neurotransmitters and chemicals that transmit messages between nerve cells. It is essential for normal brain growth and operation and also plays a major role in the production of body hormones such as serotonin, norepinephrine, and melatonin. These hormones regulate mood and the circadian or body clock. Along with vitamins B12 and B9 (folic acid), vitamin B6 helps to control levels of homocysteine in the blood. Homocysteine is an amino acid that could be linked to heart disorders.

Vitamin B6 is needed for the absorption of vitamin B12, the production of red blood cells, and cells of the immune system. Inadequate amounts of vitamin B6 is linked to heart disease, vomiting, nausea, age associated muscular deterioration, depression, premenstrual syndrome, or arthritis.

Sources of Pyridoxine can be found in sweet potato, potatoes, spinach, sunflower seeds, bananas, tuna, turkey, beef, chicken, and salmon.

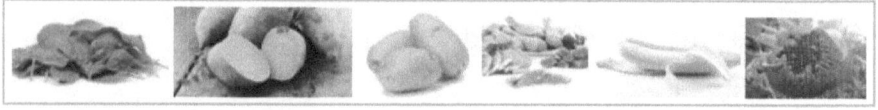

2.2.1.7. VITAMIN B7 OR H (BIOTIN)

Vitamin B7 or Biotin absorbs carbohydrates, fats, and amino acids which are the building blocks of protein. Biotin is often recommended for stronger hair and nails and it is incorporated in numerous cosmetic products designed for hair and skin. Biotin is produced by bacteria in the intestine but it cannot be stored. It can also be found in small quantities in a number of foods such as peanuts, almonds, sweet potato, eggs, onions, oats, tomatoes, carrots, walnuts, and salmon. Biotin is also vital for normal embryonic progress, making it an indispensable nutrient throughout gestation.

Deficiency in biotin is not common but lack of it results to hair loss, dry scaly skin, cracking in the corners of the mouth (cheilitis), 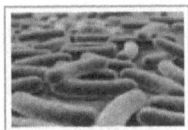 inflamed and sore tongue that is magenta in colour (glossitis), dry eyes, anorexia, lethargy, sleeplessness, and depression. People may also have to endure prolonged autoimmune diseases like Crohn's disease and require long term antibiotics and anti-seizure medications.

2.2.1.8. VITAMIN B8 (INOSITOL)

Inositol is not considered a vitamin because it is an organically occurring glucose isomer. Nevertheless, it is an indispensable nutrient for the body. Myo-inositol is biologically effective and is a significant structural element of skeletal, heart and brain tissue. Another important function of vitamin B8 is in the proper development of the liver, bone marrow cells, cholesterol transport, and in the synthesis of RNA. Inositol is essential for the body as it is needed in the process of fat and cholesterol metabolism. It acts as a mild lipotropic agent that eliminates fats from the liver and reduces blood cholesterol. Research has verified that vitamin B8 prevents symptoms of polycystic ovary syndrome (PCOS) involving infertility with major weight loss and strengthens "good" cholesterol (HDL) levels. It is used for the prevention of plaque build-up and arteriosclerosis (hardening of the arteries). It also maintains strong, healthy hair and skin and has been used to prevent and cure eczema. Some people call it a "brain food" as it works with choline in brain cell nourishment. Along with choline, vitamin B8 supports the formation of lecithin, a key building block of cell membranes that protects cells from oxidation. Inositol creates the shielding sheath around the brain which is an indispensable part of myelin that protects nerves and controls nerve transmission. Moreover, it is used in the treatment of nerve disorders as it has the ability to improve nerve function in diabetics who suffer from pain and numbness resulting from nerve deterioration. Vitamin B8 produces a soothing effect so it is also used in treating depression, panic attacks and obsessive-compulsive disorder.

Lack of vitamin B8 can result to eye anomalies, hair loss, alopecia or sparse bald headedness, memory loss, eczema, constipation, higher cholesterol levels and excess liver fat. Most of the above ailments can result to hardening and narrowing of arteries (atheriosclerosis). Inositol helps in the regeneration of the nervous system in people who suffer from multiple sclerosis, ALS, diabetic disorders, and other nervous autoimmune conditions.

Good sources for Inositol include liver, brown rice, cereals, citrus fruits, lecithin granules, beef heart, desiccated liver, wheat germ, lecithin oil, whole grain bread, soy flour, nuts, molasses, and green leafy vegetables. Inositol can also be obtained from vegetables and breakfast cereal which, in combination of phosphorous in them, form the compound known as phytic acid.

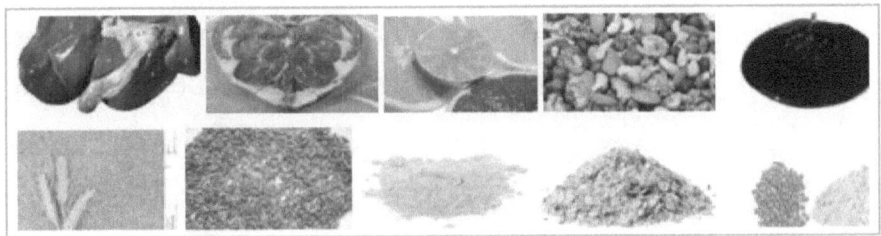

2.2.1.9. VITAMIN B9 (FOLIC ACID)

Folic acid is required in the efficient brain function which aids in maintaining proper mental and emotional well-being. It is also essential in the production of DNA and RNA (genetic material) particularly during the rapid development of cells and tissues in infancy, puberty, and gestation.

Folic acid and vitamin B12 are important for the formation and restoration of the nervous system and specifically myelin. Myelin is an electrically isolating protein-phospholipid layer that envelopes the axons of several neurons. The function of the myelin sheath is to permit impulses to be transmitted swiftly and efficiently along the nerve cells. If the myelin is damaged, the impulses slow down. This can cause syndromes such as Multiple Sclerosis (MS) and Amyotrophic Lateral Sclerosis (ALS).

Heavy drinking, bowel disease, and celiac disease could cause folic acid deficiency leads to poor growth, birth abnormalities, loss of appetite as well as anaemia. Red blood cells are created in the bone marrow and circulate within the blood system. Their life span is only four months, thus the body needs to produce more blood cells. To do so, it requires 3 vital substances namely: Iron, vitamin B12 and Folic Acid. Without them, the development of red blood cells is hampered resulting to anaemia.

Good food sources for folic acid are spinach, asparagus, broccoli, carrots, beans, peas and lentils, avocado, cauliflower, nuts such as peanuts, sunflower seeds, and flax seeds as well as almonds. It can also be obtained from fruit like papaya, oranges, grapefruits, raspberries and strawberries.

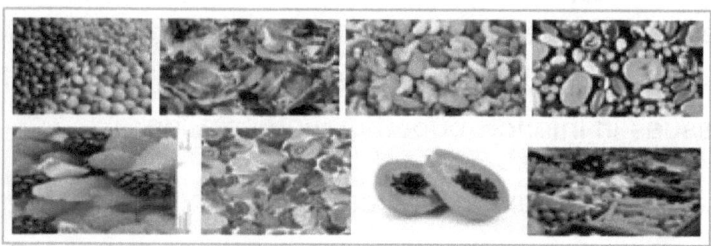

2.2.1.10. VITAMIN B10 (PABA- Para Amino Benzoic Acid)

Vitamin B10 is involved in the production of folic acid by intestinal bacteria. It is a co-enzyme in **protein metabolism** and **blood cell formation**. Vitamin B10 is important in the development of useful microorganisms in the body. It stops the bacteriostatic functions of several drugs due to its biochemical structure which is similar to sulphonamides. It is used in the treatment of irritable bowel syndrome, gastrointestinal disorders, and numerous inflammatory effects.

Similarly, PABA acts as a co-enzyme which helps in the proper use of protein by the cells. It defends the skin from free radicals which are destructive chemicals originating from contaminated air and infrared rays from the sun resulting to sunburn. PABA also aids in the treatment of skin infections like fibrotic disorder and acts as an anti-allergen on the skin. Finally, it breaks down oestrogen in the liver and delays early skin aging and greying of the hair. Deficiency of vitamin B10 can cause skin diseases, gastrointestinal disorders, inflammatory diseases, uneasiness, tetchiness, delayed growth of children, and constipation in women.

Good food sources of vitamin B10 are mushrooms, liver, molasses, eggs, yogurt, whole grains, spinach and other vegetables.

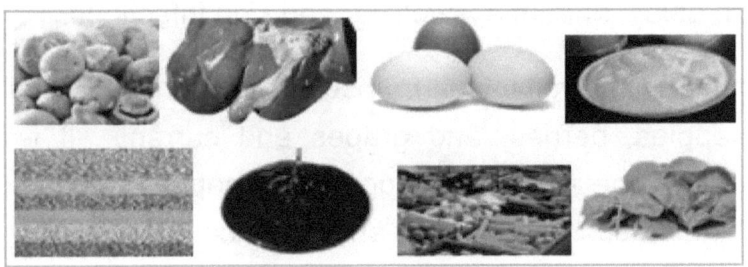

2.2.1.11. VITAMIN B11 (SALYCILIC ACID)

Salicylic acid is obtained from the metabolism of salicin, a naturally occurring compound found in the bark of several species of trees, particularly the willow, poplar, and aspen families. With its several functions in photosynthesis, ion uptake, and in transposition of plants, this ingredient aids in the growth and development of vegetation. Salicylic acid is produced naturally in the body with the support of phenylalanine amino acid. Together with vitamin B12, it plays a role in the development of RNA, DNA and red blood cells.

Vitamin B11 is an important component in the development and formation of cells from as early as the foetus phase. Growth and skin revitalization of the skin can also be achieved by using skin ointments wherein the vitamin is found thus making them effective in treating skin problems such as acne, psoriasis, warts and other skin diseases. Vitamin B11 functions as a safe anti-inflammatory agent, too, as it is a natural aspirin derived from foods. As such, it does not cause the usual adverse effects of commercially manufactured aspirin. Deficiency of this vitamin can trigger growth delay, anaemia, swelling, and skin infections.

Vitamin B11 is available in fruit such as cherries, figs, plums, kiwi, apples, berries, and grapes and currants. It is also found in vegetables like eggplants, paprika, cucumbers, zucchini, broccoli, cauliflower and liquorice.

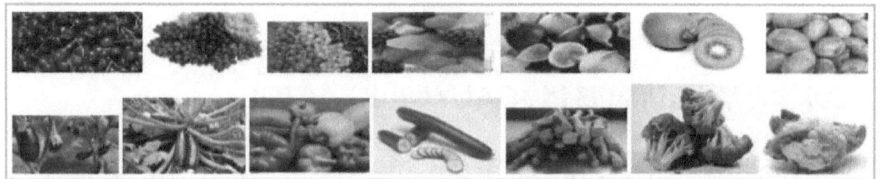

2.2.1.12. VITAMIN B12 (COBALAMIN)

Vitamin B12 is an essential element for the formation of RNA, DNA and red blood cells in the body. It is also important in the creation of certain amino acids for the appropriate function of the organism. Vitamin B12 can be produced by bacteria found in the intestinal gut. It is also beneficial in the metabolism of cells and in boosting vitality; hence some athletes are injected with it to achieve enhanced performance. As stated earlier, together with folic acid, vitamin B12 can restore the nervous system.

Insufficient amounts of this vitamin results in anaemia. Fortunately, Vitamin B12 can easily be obtained from fish, crustaceans, red meat, cereals, eggs, dairy products, shellfish, beef, and liver.

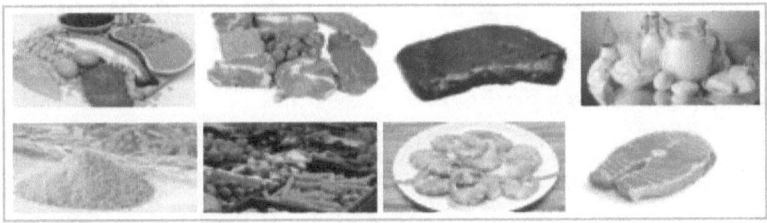

2.2.1.13. VITAMIN B13 (OROTIC ACID)

Orotic Acid was initially thought to have been part of vitamin B complex, but as it was found to be created in rich amounts by gastric flora and by a mitochondrial enzyme known as dihydroorotate dehydrogenase, it is no longer 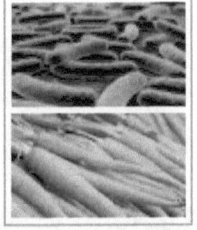 identified as such. Nevertheless, orotic acid is needed for the production of hereditary material. It may also be helpful after a heart attack so multiple sclerosis and chronic hepatitis patients can also benefit from it. However, in the presence of certain metabolic disorder, it may build up in the body, and with increased in ammonia levels, may cause orotic aciduria and academia. Vitamin B13 is mostly found in carrots.

2.2.1.14. VITAMIN B14
(XANTHOPTERIN OR METABOLITES)

Vitamin B14 is derived from wine and can be transformed by microorganisms into Folic Acid. Even though it is quite effective in the development of body cells, it is not required. Vitamin B14 offers endurance in battling anaemia and provides improvement in anti-tumour development of proteins such as pterin phosphate. Although it is not vital for formation of body cells, it is still considered significant because its absence may cause destruction of red blood cells, anaemia, pernicious anaemia, and cancerous cell development in the body.

Vitamin B14 can be found in wines and food such as eggs, meat, liver, kidney, heart, grains, yeast, and legumes.

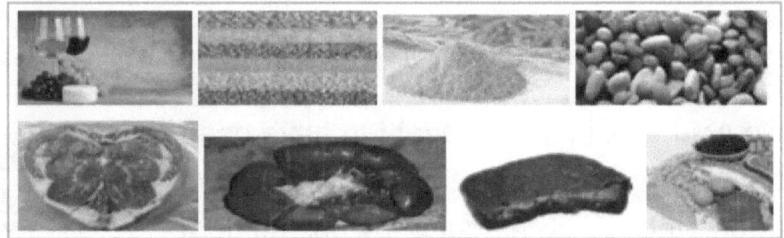

2.2.1.15. VITAMIN B15 (PANGAMIC ACID)

This organic compound defined as d-gluconodimethylamino acetic acid is also known as pangamic acid or pangamate. It helps in the formation of certain amino acids such as methionine and plays a role in the oxidation of glucose and in cell respiration. Like vitamin E, vitamin B15 may act as an antioxidant by assisting in the increase of cell life and protecting it from oxidation. Pangamic acid slightly arouses the endocrine and nervous systems and supports the detoxification procedure by improving liver function.

The former Soviet Union greatly believes in the properties of pangamic acid and its importance as a nutrient. They claim that it causes positive physiological effects that can cure an array of symptoms and illnesses. Russian researchers have proven that pangamic acid supplementation can diminish the build-up of lactic acid in athletes and thus minimizes muscle weakness and upsurges strength. Pangamic acid has been known to lower blood cholesterol, increase blood flow, and stimulate the overall oxygenation of cells and tissues. Moreover, it provides support in arteriosclerosis and hypertension. The FSU regularly uses it as treatment for alcoholism, drug dependence, and psychological problems such as old age related disorders and senility. It has also been commonly used for minimal brain damage in children, autism, and schizophrenia, heart disease and high blood pressure, diabetes, liver disease, and chemical poisonings.

Deficiency in pangamic acid can result into prolonged pain and fatigue, chronic infection leading to cancer, heart diseases, arthritis, atherosclerosis, hypertension, and cirrhosis of the liver. Finally, lack of it may cause asthma, .emphysema, alcoholism, autism, and hypoxia.

Pangamic acid can be naturally obtained from sources such as brewer yeast, whole brown rice, sesame seeds, apricot and pumpkin seeds.

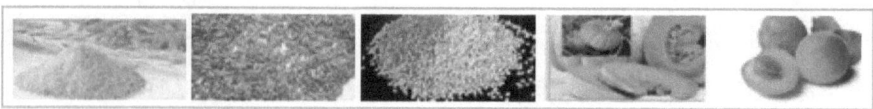

2.2.1.16. VITAMIN B16 (DIMETHYLGLYCINE)

Vitamin B16 is a derivative of the amino acid glycine. It has an equally organic structure as a water-soluble vitamin. Vitamin B16 is absorbed in the small intestine and is then further converted into useful metabolites by the liver.

Vitamin B16 behaves as a building block to DNA, amino acids, neurotransmitters and hormones. While it can invigorate the immune system and support autism treatment, epilepsy, and mitochondrial disease, vitamin B16 is not considered a vitamin since deficiency of it does not cause any harm to the body.

Vitamin B16 can be found in foods such as yeast, pumpkin seeds, apricot kernels, brewer' s sunflower seeds, and brown rice.

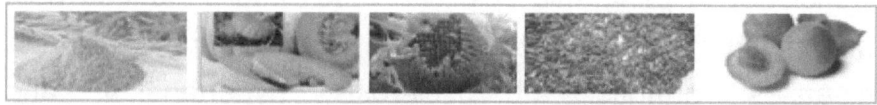

2.2.1.17. VITAMIN B17 (AMYGDALIN, LAETRILE)

Vitamin B17 can be considered as one of the very important vitamins. Even though there are still controversies about it not being a vitamin, some believe that not recognising it as such disregards its many benefits.   There have also been false investigations that stated that amygdalin does not work but nothing could be farther from the truth. Neither chemotherapeutics nor anything biochemical can duplicate the effects of vitamin B17. It belongs to the group of nitrilosides which are an extensive group of water-soluble, non-toxic, sugary compounds, obtained from numerous plants.   They commonly termed as beta-cyanophoric glycosides.

On page 56 of G. Edward Griffin book *World without Cancer*, he emphasizes why nitriloside is really a vitamin. Amygdalin is made up of four molecules: 2 sugars, 1 benzaldehyde and 1 cyanide. The cyanide is basically what justifies the dispute around this vitamin particularly in regards to cancer malignancy treatments. Typical cells have an enzyme called rhodanase. This enzyme disables the cyanide molecule of the laetrile compound. Cancer cells do not have this enzyme. More specifically what they do possess is beta-glucosidase which is an enzyme that discharges the cyanide, which then destroys the cancer cells.

According to his book Griffin states that, vitamin-B17 originates from bitter almond, apricot, blackthorn, cherry, nectarine, peach, plum, grass, maize, sorghum, millet, cassava, linseed, apples seeds, and several other foods that have commonly been excluded from the list of options of contemporary cultures. If appropriate nourishment is not present in one's diet and there is an excess in the consumption of bad carbohydrates and fats, the deficiency in Vitamin B17 could encourage cancer development.

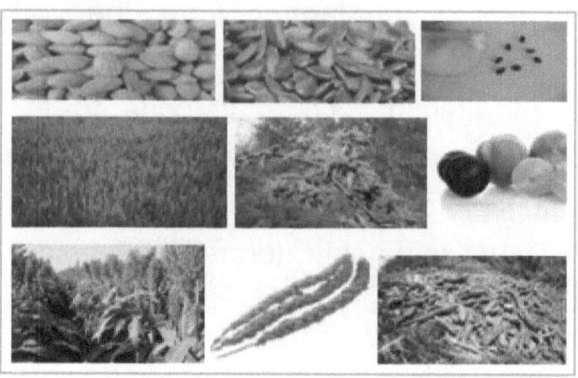

2.2.2. VITAMIN C (ASCORBIC ACID)

Vitamin C is a well-known compound but sad to say, not many people are aware of its actual properties. Vitamin C is essential for the development of collagen, a protein required to effectively grow skin, tendons, ligaments and blood vessels. It can restore injuries, mend, and preserve cartilage, bones, and teeth and it is one of the best easily available antioxidants. Vitamin C is capable of cleansing our system from free radicals. Free radicals and antioxidants will later be discussed in detail in ___ section.

Another important function of Vitamin C is to protect the fat-soluble vitamins A and E, as well as fatty acids from oxidation. Besides forming free radicals oxidation, it fights and alleviates scurvy disease. It can be valuable in the management of iron inadequacy and it aids in increasing its absorption. Vitamin C can also be vital in tackling anaemia, particularly megaloblastic anaemia. If vitamin C is not present in adequate amount, it can cause scurvy, common cold, capillary brittleness, asthma, gingivitis, gout, musculoskeletal damages, and recurrent allergies.

Some facts to know about Vitamin C:

- Unlike other animals, humans, primates, and guinea pigs, cannot produce vitamin C naturally in themselves. They can only get it from outside sources such as in fruit and vegetables such as in papaya, bell peppers, broccoli, Brussels sprouts, strawberries, pineapple, oranges, kiwi, cantaloupe, cauliflower, grapefruit, parsley, and lemon among others.

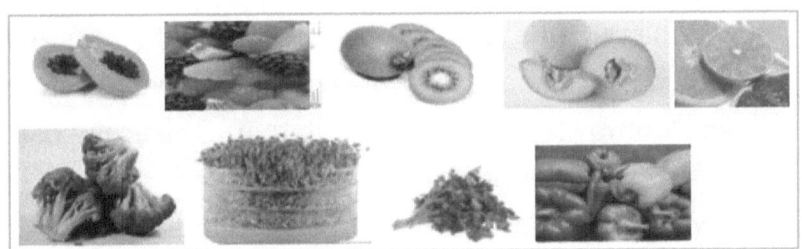

- Smokers are not able to absorb vitamin C in the same amounts as people who do not smoke.

- Scarcity of vitamin C is accountable for the infections that can trigger heart attacks, strokes, and other associated circulatory syndromes. How is that possible? As mentioned earlier, vitamin C can only be acquired from food. Therefore, inappropriate diets, as well smoking, can lead to the lack of vitamin C in the body. One of the vital elements for the development of the cardiac system is collagen which is created by vitamin C along with other substances. Without enough collagen, the vessels cannot be maintained properly and minute ruptures begin to appear in the blood vessels. How does the body work to defend the blood vessels? It deposits CHOLESTEROL on the ruptures. However, it may sometimes happen that the body deposits more cholesterol than necessary to seal the ruptured vessels. This may result to building up of plaques and cause the hardening or narrowing of the blood vessels. This process may lead to all the diseases stated above.

- How can vitamin C fight cancer? Cancer cells have the capacity to captivate glucose, iron, and copper. Since Vitamin C has a composition similar to the glucose molecule, cancer cells which are sometimes referred to as "dump cells" mistake Vitamin C as glucose and absorb it. With iron and copper present within cancerous cells, vitamin C reacts with these metals and forms Hydrogen Peroxide, a chemical used on external lesions that produces white foam. This substance can demolish the carcinogenic cells. More information or details on this can be obtained from Holistic Health Practitioners. Vitamin C is a very important to the body should not be overlooked. It must remain a top priority of everyday nutritional intakes.

CONCLUSION

Vitamins play vital role in sustaining health and providing people with the nutrients necessary for a healthy life. The power of raw food lies on its simplicity. By consuming fresh raw food that is unprocessed and pure, people are assured of obtaining proper nourishment while being in harmony with nature's purpose and their bodies' needs. This is the best way to get the utmost benefits from vitamins in the form and manner nature intended them to be. There is indeed beauty in the natural and simple so keep it that way.

Chapter 2

MINERALS

Just like vitamins, minerals help your body grow, develop, regenerate, and stay healthy. Minerals make up for about 4% of the human body and must be taken by food. There are 103 known minerals and at least 18 of them are necessary for good health. They help enzymes to react properly, maintain the pH balance in the body, support the transfer of nutrients across cell membranes, maintain the proper functions of nervous, bone and muscle system, aids tissue growth, and for the overall support of the body. Minerals are divided in to two categories: the Macro-minerals and the Trace-minerals. Macro is derived from the Greek word which means 'large'. That means that although the body needs both categories of minerals, it needs macro-minerals in larger quantities daily.

MACRO-MINERALS

In this group belongs, calcium, phosphorus, magnesium, sodium, potassium, chloride, and sulphur.

1.1 CALCIUM (Ca)

Calcium is responsible for healthy bones and teeth. Deficiency of this mineral can cause osteoporosis and other bone related diseases. It plays a vital role in the proper muscle contraction. Food sources for calcium are dairy products, vegetables such as broccoli, rhubarb, kum quat, many other fruits as well as dried figs and apricots.

1.2 PHOSPHORUS (Ph)

Phosphorus is an essential component of living systems and is found in the nervous tissue, bones, teeth, and cell protoplasm. The main function of phosphorus is in the formation of bones and teeth. It also plays an important role in how the body metabolizes carbohydrates, protein, and fats for the growth and in the maintenance and repairs of cells and tissues. Phosphorus also helps the body make ATP, a molecule the body uses to store energy. It helps the B vitamins for normal heartbeat, nerve signalling, muscle contraction and kidney function. Phosphorous can be found in seeds, dairy products, meat, fish, beans and lentils.

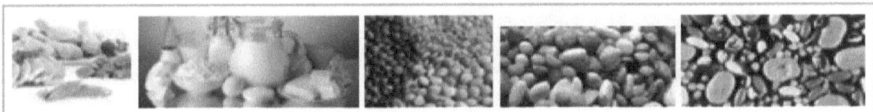

1.3 MAGNESIUM (Mg)

According to the Institute of Medicine and Lippincott Williams & Wilkins; 2012, magnesium is a co-factor in more than 300 enzyme systems that regulate diverse biochemical reactions in the body, including protein synthesis, muscle and nerve function, blood glucose control and blood regulation. It is required for energy production, oxidative prhosphrylation and glycolysis. It contributes to the structural development of bone and is required for DNA and RNA synthesis. Magnesium is vital for the transport of calcium and potassium across cell membrane, which is important in nerve tissue conduction, muscle contraction and proper heartbeat. Since the kidneys cannot excrete Magnesium through urine, therefore deficiency is rare. However, in such cases as chronic alcoholism and uses of medicine pills, deficiency of this mineral may occur. Foods highest in magnesium are nuts, seeds, dark chocolate, fish, legumes, lentils, whole grains, dried fruits and fresh fruits.

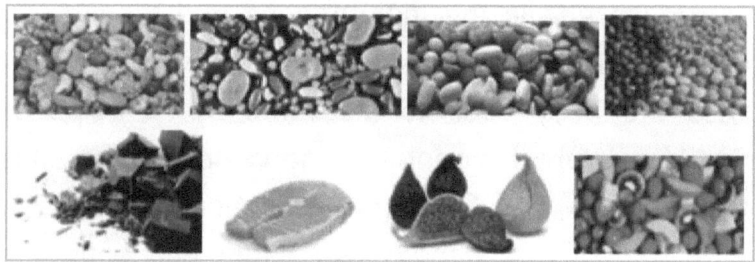

1.4 SODIUM (Na)

Sodium is a very important electrolyte and ion found in the extracellular fluid. It plays an essential role in the osmoregulation and fluid maintenance within the human body. It helps in enzyme operations, muscle contractions, and improves the performance of heart and nervous system. Sodium also enhances glucose absorption.

Vegetables like celery, carrots, spinach, broccoli, peppers and beets are good sources of sodium. Fruits also contain sufficient amount of it. However, avoid the table salt which contains 40% of Sodium. Table salt is not a natural source of sodium and can harm your arteries and veins. The table salt cannot be diluted and it scuffs the vessels while passing through them. Please see the section on vitamin C. But you can use instead Himalayan salt which contains 84 natural minerals or Celtic salt and are healthy.

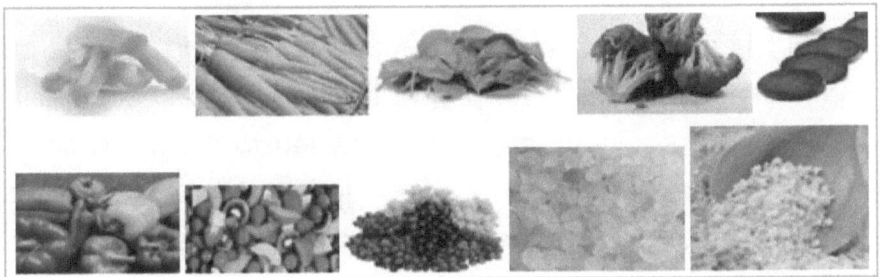

1.5 POTASSIUM (K)

Potassium relaxes the vessels from pressure, prevents heart and kidneys from any disorder, 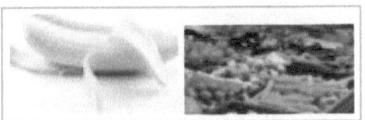 reduces anxiety and stress, and maintains muscles, metabolism, water balance, electrolytic functions, and nervous system. Fruits, especially banana, and vegetables contain sufficient Potassium to meet the daily amount required.

1.6 CHLORIDE (CI)

Chloride is an essential element of digestive stomach liquids. It plays an important role in the balance of body fluids.

Chloride can be found in grains, vegetables and fruits in sufficient amount to meet the daily requirement for it.

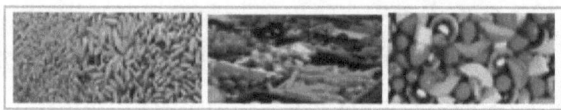

1.7 SULPHUR (S)

Sulphur is a nutrient compound found in all living organisms and it is absolutely vital for proper health. It is responsible in providing the sufficient amount of oxygen to the living cells. In the old days, farmers used to apply animal manure to crops to enrich the soil naturally with high levels of sulphur. Unfortunately, today's industrialized farming methods strip the soil of sulphur. Even the food itself loses sulphur through processing because when the mineral is converted from crystal to powder, it loses 85% of its effectiveness by, refrigeration, dehydration and cooking.

Sulphur can improve the resistance to illness and maintains muscle flexibility as well. It can reduce inflammations, prevents osteoporosis, as well as degenerative nervous diseases. It can increase blood circulation and detoxifies at a cellular level including heavy metals. It helps the pancreas produce enough amount of insulin in the body. With vitamin C, sulphur is responsible for collagen building that keeps vessels and skin young and healthy. It acts like an anti-parasitic agent; it has antagonist receptors with parasites that prevents them from attaching to the intestinal wall. It also prevents cancer.

Scar tissue, wrinkles, damaged skin, lung dysfunction, diabetes, sore joints and muscles, ulcers, migraine headaches, allergic reactions, candida albicans, infections, high cholesterol, and diverticulitis are the main symptoms of deficiency.

The good food sources for sulphur are cruciferous vegetables such as broccoli, cauliflower, Brussels sprouts, etc. Allium vegetables, such as garlic, onions, leeks and chives also contain organosulfur compounds. Other good sources of sulphur are food rich in protein such as meat, fish, dairy products and especially eggs that have 0.2 milligrams of sulphur.

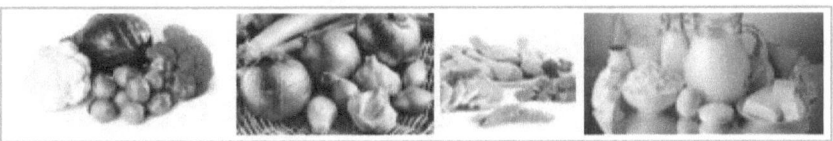

2. 0 TRACE-MINERALS

Trace minerals are a group of minerals that the body needs in very small amounts. The recommended dietary allowance (RDA) for most vitamins and minerals is 800 to 1,200 milligrams per day. For trace minerals, the RDA averages between 0.2 milligrams and 15 milligrams per day, depending on the mineral. Among the most important of the trace minerals are iron, copper, zinc, selenium, manganese, molybdenum, iodine, chromium and fluoride.

2.1 IRON (Fe)

Iron is essential for the production of haemoglobin and red blood cells. It plays a key role in growth and development of humans and animals. Since it is an oxygen carrier, is very important in red blood cells and muscles (myoglobin) functioning. It also helps in the immune system and regulates body temperature. It provides oxygen to the brain for proper concentration.

Iron deficiency can lead to conditions like iron deficiency anaemia, chronic anaemia, cough, and pre-dialysis anaemia. In some animals, like in pigs, piglets from the 2nd day of birth, they must take exogenous iron because there is a possibility for them to develop anaemia and die.

Iron is found in red meat, egg yolks, dark leafy greens like spinach, dried fruit, liver, beans, lentils in general and artichokes. Iron is better absorbed with vitamin C.

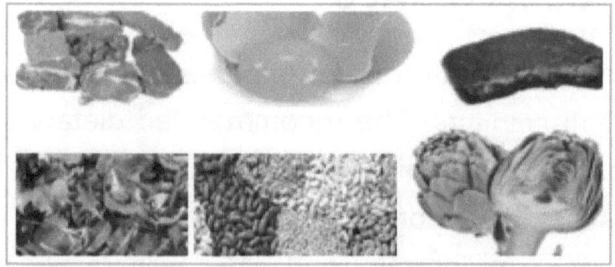

2.2 COPPER (Cu)

Copper is the third mineral most essential for growth and health. It helps in red blood cell formation by increasing the absorption of iron. It plays a significant role in the formation of haemoglobin, myelin and elastin. It ensures proper functioning of the thyroid gland, prevents premature aging, and improves immune system. Copper reacts with more than 40 different enzymes in the body for proper functioning of metabolism.

Deficiency of copper may lead to anaemia, arthritis, degeneration of nervous system, osteoporosis, thyroid disorders, low body temperature, low resistance to infections and others. Since copper cannot be manufactured by the body, it must be taken from exogenous food sources like meat, seafood, whole grains, sesame and sunflower seeds, cashews, soybeans, lentils and legumes, almonds, avocados, mushrooms and walnuts.

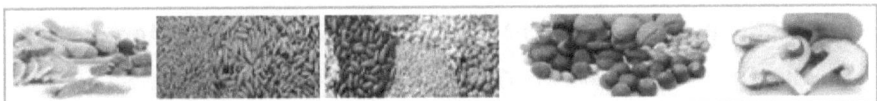

2.3 ZINC (Zn)

Zinc can be found in food such as seafood, meat, wheat germ, spinach, pumpkin and squash seeds, nuts, cocoa and dark chocolate, beans and mushrooms. Zinc earns its stripes by promoting immune function to fight illness, supporting healthy cell growth and development, and ensuring a proper sense of taste and smell.

Zinc is especially important for men because of its role in maintaining prostate health, testosterone levels and overall sexual health. But since our bodies do not produce zinc naturally, a daily intake of it is recommended to ensure healthy levels of this critical mineral.

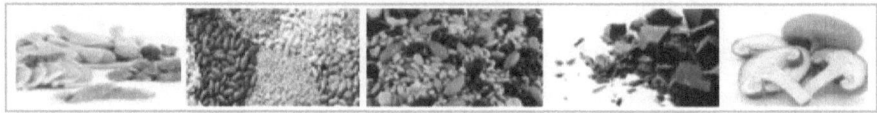

2.4 SELENIUM (Se)

Selenium is found mostly in liver, kidneys, pancreas, testes, and spleen. This mineral helps to fight free radicals that are harmful to the body. It acts as an antioxidant and is essential for maintenance of a healthy body. Several research studies demonstrated the benefits of selenium supplementation in treating autoimmune thyroid conditions and general thyroid dysfunctions which is the battery of our hormonal balance. Selenium can be found in abundance in Brazil nuts, seeds, fish and meat. Take 5 Brazil nuts daily and you have more than enough of selenium that body requires.

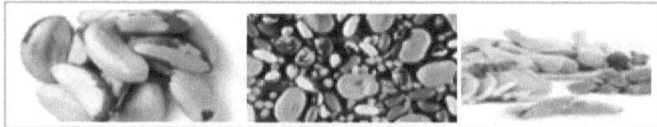

2.5 MANGANESE (Mn)

Manganese plays an essential role in the metabolism of food intake, helps in the normal functioning of nervous system, and works as an antioxidant. It also helps in the formation of hormones like thyroxin and sex hormones. Manganese can be found high in seafood, nuts and seeds. It also can be found in cloves, spinach, pineapple, brown rice, rye, soybeans and others.

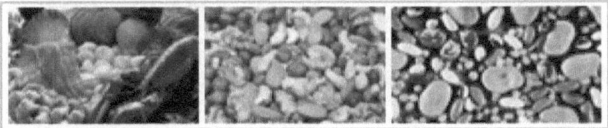

2.6 MOLYBDENUM (Mo)

Molybdenum is an essential mineral in breaking down proteins and other substances, as well as in protecting the cells from free radicals. Overdose can lead to poor digestibility of copper and then anaemia may occur. It could be found in beans, soybeans, nuts and dairy products.

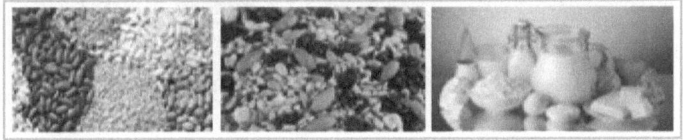

2.7 IODINE (I)

Iodine rich foods include seaweed (especially kelp), beans, organic cultured yogurt, organic non-sugared cranberry juice or fresh cranberries, unprocessed Himalayan salt, and fresh organic strawberries. These foods are among the top choices for iodine to keep your thyroid hormone production high. This helps in the optimal utilization of calories, thereby preventing its storage as excess fat. Other benefits of iodine are removing toxins from the body and helping the system to utilize various minerals like calcium and silicon.

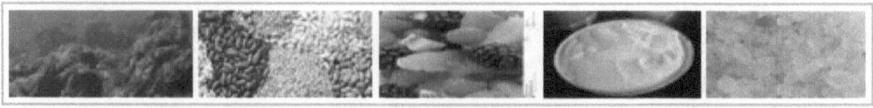

2.8 CHROMIUM (Cr)

Chromium is very important for the synthesis of proteins, fats, and cholesterol. It also plays an important role in the metabolism of glucose thus making it one of the nutrients necessary for diabetics. This mineral is usually supplemented in the form of chromium picolinate. Food rich in chromium are **brewer's yeast**, coffee, tea, **cereals**, potatoes, **peas**, **oysters**, **rye**, **thyme**, processed meats, **whole grains**, and beer.

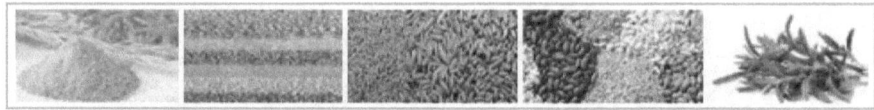

2.9 FLUORIDE (F)

When fluoride is taken with food, it is naturally converted to calcium fluoride and strengthens the teeth and bones. This mineral occurs naturally as a sodium fluoride in the ocean, so most seafood contains fluoride. Generally, all the fresh food and water contain 0.01-0.1 ppm of fluoride, which is more than enough for our health.

Unfortunately, most processed water and food contain large amounts of fluoride which can lead to fluorosis. Even foods made with mechanically deboned meat (e.g nuggets) contain elevated levels of fluoride due to the contamination from bone particles that occurs during the mechanical deboning process. Fluorosis is a condition that affects the teeth and bones. It is caused by overexposure to fluoride. Fluorosis can cause osteoporosis, osteoarthritis, arthritis, rheumatoid arthritis. Fluoride may also damage connective tissue, brain, and testicles. Also be careful from drinking water containing extra fluoride.

Chapter 3

VITAMINS

Enzymes are large biological molecules produced by living organism and act as catalysts to bring biochemical transformations in all parts of the body. They are responsible for the thousands of metabolic processes that sustain life. The most striking characteristics of enzymes are their *catalytic power* and *specificity* (only when the right enzyme finds the right substrate can biochemical reactions occur). Nearly all enzymes are proteins. Each enzyme is made of between a hundred and upwards of a million amino acids placed like pearls on a string. Each amino acid is bonded to the next by chemical bonds. The vast majority of enzymes are made of only 20 different kinds of amino acid. When using chemicals, most industries have production waste that presents a threat to nature. Enzymes can do the same job at lesser cost without threat to the environment. Enzymes are a part of nature and are therefore fully biodegradable.

Enzymes have three major functions. The first is to increase the rate of a reaction. Most cellular reactions occur about a million times faster than they would in the absence of an enzyme. Second, most enzymes act specifically with only one reactant (called a **substrate**) to produce products. The third and most remarkable characteristic is that enzymes are regulated from a state of low activity to high activity and vice versa.

Enzymes are commonly named by adding a suffix "-ase" to the root name of the substrate molecule it is acting upon, like lipase which catalyzes the hydrolysis of lipids. A few enzymes discovered before this naming system was devised are known by common names. Examples are pepsin, trypsin, and chymotrypsin which catalyzes the hydrolysis of proteins.

There are six broad groups of enzymes.

1. Oxidase or Dehydrogenase – oxidation/reduction reactions

2. Transferase – transfer

3. Hydrolase – hydrolysis reactions

4. Lyase – addition to double bonds or its reverse

5. Isomerase – isomerization reactions

6. Ligase / Synthetase – formation of bond with ATP cleavage

Enzymes can be produced naturally by our system. But there are some foods containing a good amount of enzymes which helps in the 6 processes mentioned above. These high enzyme foods are: **papaya** (contains papain – proteolytic ability, ie brakes down the proteins into amino-acids.); **pineapple** (contains bromelain – also proteolytic enzyme); **sprouts** (are the seeds of many different types of grains. These foods are packed with nutrients and may contain more than 100 times more enzymes than fruits and vegetables. Sprouts are the most concentrated with active enzymes when they are germinated); **nuts and seeds** (contain lipase for the hydrolysis of lipids); **and other fruits and vegetables** (mostly contain amylase for the enzymatic hydrolysis of carbohydrates). These foods can deliver their enzymes in their raw stage only. Enzymes are very sensitive to heat.

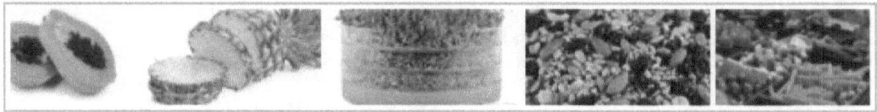

Chapter 4

FREE RADICALS

What makes us old or what keeps us young, is a matter of the amount of free radicals in our organism. The more we have of these free radicals, the faster we become older. In order to understand what free radicals are, we have to learn about atoms, molecules, protons, neutrons and electrons which what we are made of basically.

What are atoms? Atoms are the basic building blocks of matter that make up everyday objects. It is true that everything is made up of atoms, even we, humans and animals. There are until now, around 90 naturally occurring kids of atoms and many other chemically occurring kinds. Now, atoms are made out of three basic particles: the Protons (which carry positive charge), the Neutrons (which carry no charge), and the Electrons (which carry negative charge). Protons and Neutrons join together and form the nucleus of the atom, while Electrons circle the nucleus.

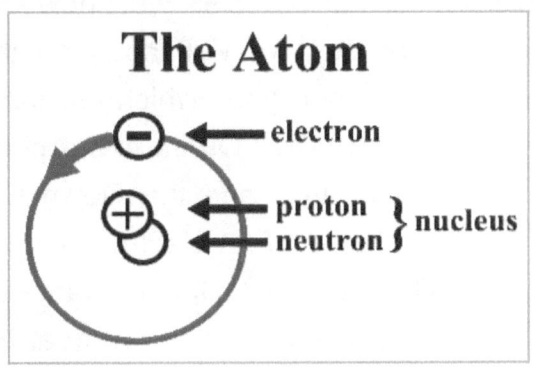

The Atom

electron

proton } nucleus
neutron

Depending on how many protons are together, they form the molecular element. For example if we take a look in a periodic table, it starts with Hydrogen. The Hydrogen consists of 1 proton. Have in mind that the number of protons are always the same as the number of electrons. Neutrons determine the atomic mass of the element. For example, there are 29 protons (and electrons) and 34 neutrons in the element Copper (Cu). In periodic table Copper is in 29th place, so its atomic number is 29, but its atomic mass is 63.

What are Proton, Neutron and Electron made of? I will go deeper to show you how we are made. You will be surprised!

An elementary or fundamental particle is the particle that does not have a substructure so it cannot be split further into smaller particles. So Electron is the one but what about the proton and neutron? They are made up of smaller particles called quarks.

Quarks are fundamental particles made of energies holding together and according to their spin; they have a positive or negative fractional charge. Quarks are the fundamental building blocks on all the particles we know of. They are divided into six kinds. But we will focus on the naturally occurring and most common ones which are the Up Quarks and the Down Quarks. The Up Quark has a charge of +2/3 of the charge of an electron and the Down Quark has a charge of -1/3 of the charge of an electron. Thus a Proton is made up of 2 Up Quarks and 1 Down Quark. In maths we have **+2/3 + +2/3 + -1/3 = 3/3** which is equal to 1. That is why a proton has a positive charge. Now what about Neutron? Neutron is made up of 1 Up Quark and 2 Down Quarks. So is **+2/3 + -1/3 + -1/3 = 0** charge. That is why we call it Neutron, because of the neutral. These Quarks are holding together with electromagnetic forces and the whole mass forms Protons and Neutrons.

Electrons are also fundamental building blocks of which the universe is made of. Together with Protons and Neutrons they form the Atom which is responsible in building organic and inorganic matters. The Potential Energy of electrons alone is zero. When it comes closer to a nucleus of the atom, then the energy becomes lower than zero and since it is lower, the charge is negative. From this time, it is controlled by the nucleus (because of the positive charge of protons) and is moving around it. Let's learn some definitions in order to understand further about free radicals.

What is a pair of electrons? A pair of electrons consists of electrons that occupy the same orbital but have opposite spins. The word 'orbital' refers to the Molecular Orbital (MO) and in chemistry, is used to describe the region where an electron orbits around the atom. See the blue orbital in picture above. So logically, an unpaired electron consists of just one electron that occupies alone, one Molecular Orbital. An unpaired electron is **unusual** in both organic and inorganic chemistry. In organic chemistry is called 'radical'.

Free Radicals are atoms or molecules with unpaired electrons in the outermost bonding orbital and are likely to take part in chemical reactions. Electrons prefer to be in pairs and when an electron is alone in its orbital, it will try to take an electron from another atom to become more stable. When the other atom loses its electron it tries on its turn to steal an electron from another atom, often resulting in a dangerous chain reaction. Free radicals can cause damage to our cells but they also play an important role in a number of biological processes, such as the intracellular killing of bacteria by white blood cells and some cell signalling processes. Targets of free radicals include all kind of molecules in the body. The major ones are lipids, proteins, and nucleic acids.

The most important types of free radicals are the radical derivatives of oxygen better known as Reactive Oxygen Species (ROS). When an apple slice becomes brown, when fish becomes rancid, or a cut on our skin is raw and inflamed, all of these result from a natural process called **oxidation**. These are: oxygen in its singlet state ($1O_2$), triplet state ($3O_2$), superoxide anion, hydroxyl radical, nitric oxide, peroxinitrine, hypochlorous acid, hydrogen peroxide, alkoxyl radical and the peroxyl radical. I just mention them for those who are interested looking further and learn about these names.

Catalysts: almost all metals can be free radicals. Most of them have unpaired electron in their outer orbital and can be easily susceptible. Even Iron and Copper which have paired electrons in there outer orbital, can easily lose one of their electrons.

Why do we have free radicals in our body? Where do they come? We cannot completely get rid of free radicals because our body naturally produce some. For example, we need chemical reactions producing free radicals in our organism if we want to stay alive, or our immune system produces free radicals to fight off microorganisms and diseases. Not all free radicals are bad but they become problems when the amount of free radicals is greater than the body can handle, resulting to serious damage to the molecules building our organism. Some environmental factors that increase free radical production are:

1. Daily emotional and physical stress
2. Ozone depletion
3. Air pollutants
4. Smoke
5. Radiation
6. Industrial Chemicals
7. Processed foods
8. Drugs

What can be caused to organism by ROS Free Radicals? A growing number of diseases and disorders have been linked either directly or indirectly to these reactive species such as:

1. Deterioration noted in aging
2. Atherosclerosis (heart disease, stroke)
3. Brain disorders (ischemic brain injury, aluminium toxicity, Alzheimer disease, neurotoxins)

4. Cancer

5. Cardiac Myopathy

6. Chronic Granulomatous Disease

7. Diabetes Mellitus

8. Eye Disorders (macular degeneration, cataracts)

9. Inflammatory Disorders

10. Iron Overload

11. Lung Disorders (asbestosis, oxygen toxicity, emphysema)

12. Nutritional Deficiencies

13. Radiation Injury

14. Reperfusion Injury

15. Rheumatoid Arthritis

16. Skin Disorders (solar radiation, burns, contact dermatitis, bloom syndrome)

17. Toxic State (xenobiotics like smoke, metal ions like Niger, Copper and Iron)

How can our body fight free radicals? Mother Nature provides thousands of antioxidants in various amounts in fruits, vegetables, whole grains, nuts and legumes. Antioxidants are described in detail in chapter 5.

Chapter 5

ANTIOXIDANTS

While free radicals are unstable molecules, antioxidants, on the other hand, are low-weight molecules that are stable enough to donate an electron to a violent free radical and neutralize it. Smart yeah!!? And they inhibit the chain reaction you have learned in chapter 2, before tissues are damaged. Some of these antioxidants like glutathione, ubiquinol and uric acid, are produced during normal metabolism in the body [1]. Lighter antioxidants are found in the diet. But the main nutrients mostly responsible for the job to fight and neutralize free radicals are vitamins such as A, B complex, C and E mentioned in chapter 1.

Antioxidants have different actions separated in 4 levels:

LEVEL 1: Here are the preventive antioxidants. These antioxidants suppress the formation of free radicals. How? Some antioxidants can reduce hydroperoxides and hydrogen peroxide beforehand to alcohols and water respectively, without generation of free radicals and some proteins sequester metal ions. Antioxidants that are known to decompose lipid hydroperoxides to corresponding alcohols are: a) Glutathione Peroxidase, b) Glutathione-s-transferase, c) Phospholipid Hydroperoxide Glutathione Peroxidase

(PHGPX). Antioxidants known to reduce Hydrogen Peroxide to water are: a) Glutathione Peroxidase and b) Catalase.

LEVEL 2: Here are the antioxidants that scavenge the active free radicals to suppress and break the chain reactions. Here, the antioxidants are separated in hydrophilic, such as, vitamin C, uric acid, bilirubin, albumin and thiols. And lipophilic scavenging antioxidants, such as vitamin E and ubiquinol.

LEVEL 3: Here are the repair and *de novo* antioxidants. These antioxidants are capable of recognizing, degrading, and removing oxidatively modified proteins and prevent the accumulation of oxidized proteins. They are found in cytosol and in the mitochondria of mammalian cells and are the proteolytic enzymes, proteinases, proteases and peptidases. Glycosylases and nucleases also play an important role against oxidative damage, to the DNA repair systems.

LEVEL 4: Here involves the mechanisms of formation and transport of the appropriate antioxidant to the right site, after the signalisation of the production and reactions of free radicals. It is called Adaptation. [2]

TYPES OF ANTIOXIDANTS

All antioxidants exist in the intracellular and extracellular environment to detoxify ROS explained in chapter 3. They are separated to enzymatic and non-enzymatic.

A] ENZYMATIC

Here, cells are protected against oxidative stress by these enzymatic antioxidants and give reactions such as converting free radicals to give water.

SUPEROXIDE DISMUTASE

SuperOxide Dismutase (SOD) is a class of closely related enzymes that catalyze the breakdown of superoxide anion into Oxygen (O_2) and Hydrogen Peroxide (H_2O_2). [3]

There are 3 major families of SOD depending on the metal cofactors:

a) Cu/Zn (binding both Copper and Zinc)

b) Fe/Mn (binding Iron or Manganese)

c) Ni (binding Nickel) [4]

CATALASE

This is a common enzyme found in nearly all living organisms exposed to oxygen where it functions to catalyze the decomposition of Hydrogen Peroxide to water and oxygen. [5]

GLUTATHIONE SYSTEMS

Here belongs glutathione reductase, glutathione peroxidase and glutathione-s-transferase. For example, glutathione peroxidase with its 4 Selenium cofactors can catalyze the breakdown of hydrogen peroxide and organic hydroperoxides, while glutathione-s-transferase can catalyze lipid peroxides.

B] NON-ENZYMATIC

VITAMIN C (ASCORBIC ACID)

As explained in chapter 1, while most other animals can produce ascorbic acid in their bodies, it cannot be synthesized in humans and must be taken from his diet. Ascorbic acid is a reducing agent and can reduce and neutralize ROS like Hydrogen Peroxide.

GLUTATHIONE

It is a cysteine-containing peptide found in most forms of aerobic life. In its cysteine part, there is the thiol group, a reducing agent that can be reversibly oxidized and reduced. So in other words, glutathione can be an enzymatic as well as a non-enzymatic antioxidant and because of its high concentration and central role in maintaining the cell's red-ox state, it is one of the most important cellular antioxidants. [6]

MELATONIN

Melatonin, known chemically as Nacetyl-5-methoxytryptamine, is a naturally occurring hormone found in animals and in some other living organisms, including algae. [7] Melatonin once oxidized, cannot be reduced to its former state because it forms several stable end-products upon reacting with free radicals. Therefore, it has been referred to as a terminal or suicidal antioxidant. [8] This is why it does not undergo red-ox cycling like other antioxidants.

VITAMIN E (TOCOPHEROL AND TOCOTRIENOL)

As mentioned in chapter 1, vitamin E is a fat soluble vitamin with antioxidant properties. It has a set of 8 related tocopherols and tocotrienols but the most important of these is the a-tocopherol which protects membranes from oxidation by reacting with lipid radicals produced in the lipid peroxidation chain reaction. [9]

URIC ACID

According to Michael Rizen, MD, Internal Medicine, Uric Acid is the most abundant liquid antioxidant in the body and count for as much as two thirds of all free radical scavenging capacity in the blood. Uric acid may be able form crystals that wind up in the fluid in joints. Because urate is present in high concentrations in plasma and seems particularly efficient at inactivating 2 very powerful oxidants, HO and

HOGI, this substance can be assumed to be as a potent scavenger in vivo.

SOURCES OF NATURALLY OCCURRING ANTIOXIDANTS

- Vegetables like potatoes, spinach, broccoli and olive
- Legumes
- Fruits like berries, cherries, citrus, prunes and tomatoes
- Green teas
- Wheat sprout is the strongest antioxidant
- Purified Water
- Indian Medicinal Plants listed in table.

Indian Medicinal Plants [10]

LATIN NAMES	AYURVEDIC NAMES
Acacia catechu	Kair
Aegle marmelos	Bengal quince, Bel
Allium cepa	Onion
Allium sativum	Garlic, lahasuna
Aloe vera	Indian aloe
Amomum subulatum	Greater cardamom
Andrographis paniculata	Kiryat
Asparagus recemosus	Shatavari
Azadirachta indica	Neem, Nimba

Bacopa monniera	Brahmi
Butea monosperma	Palas, Dhak
Camellia sinensis	Green tea
Cinnamomum verum	Cinnamon
Cinnamomum tamala	Tejpat
Curcma longa	Turmeric haridra
Emblica officinalis	Indian gooseberry
Glycyrrhiza glapra	Yashtimudhu
Hemidesmus charantia	Bitter gourd
Murraya koenigii	Curry leaf
Nigella sativa	Black cumin
Ocimumu sanctum	Holy basil, Tusil
Obnosma echioides	Ratanjyot
Picrorrhiza hurroa	Katuka
Plumbago zeylancia	Chitrak
Sesamum indicum	Indian Sesame
Sida cordifolia	Flannel Weed
Spirulina fusiformis	Alga
Swertia decussata	Kadu
Syzigium cumini	Jamun
Terminalia ariuna	Arjun
Terminalia bellarica	Beheda
Tinospora cordifolia	Heart leaved moonseed, guduchi
Trgonella foenum-graecium	Fenugreek
Withania somifera	Winter cherry
Zingiber officinalis	Ginger

I hope I fulfilled your needs about getting familiar to what you need to eat and avoid in order to have a healthy life.

ABOUT THE AUTHOR

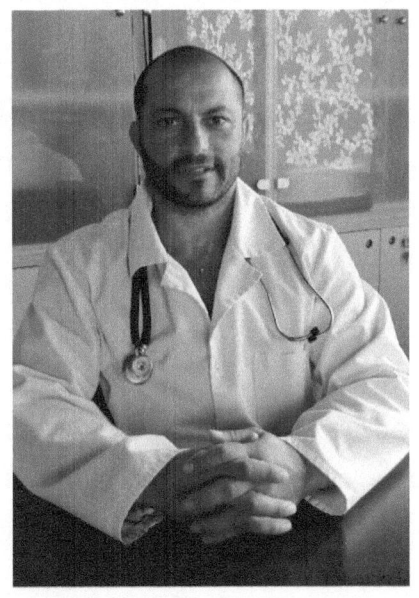

Dr. Neophytos Neophytou, or simply Dr. Neo, is a multi-faceted man who is successful in the many endeavours he engages in. He is a businessman, an author, a sportsman, a family physician, a veterinary surgeon, and a holistic practitioner rolled into one.

His career as a veterinary doctor started in 2005 when he earned his diploma in Veterinary Medicine from the Agricultural University of Wroclaw, Poland. Five years later, he became a full-pledge veterinary surgeon upon completion of his Post Graduate course in Veterinary Surgery in the same university. However, his love for animals started much earlier during his youth when his family put up a pig farm business.

Dr. Neo's concern for the health and welfare of animals went beyond animals to include the whole humanity. This led him to further his studies by enrolling at the College of Naturophatic Medicine UK via the Neo-Hippocrates Natural Therapies in Cyprus.

In 2014, he earned his two diplomas both for Naturophatic and Homeopathic Medicines from the Neo-Hippocrates Natural Therapies in Cyprus. In the same year, besides taking up Energy Healing courses in Cyprus, he also studied Electromagnetic Waves Diagnosis and Healing at the Deta Elis Russian Institute and MLM.

Equipped with all these knowledge, Dr. Neo embarked in his life-long dream of caring both for humans and animals as a veterinarian, a family physician, and a holistic health practitioner.

Inspired by the holistic principle that humans' needs were not limited to their physical health, Dr. Neo decided to address their economic necessities as well. However, he believed that giving dole-outs was not the answer. He thought that helping them to fend for themselves was a more lasting and empowering assistance. This was when he decided to put up his networking business which gave others the opportunity to improve their lives.

It was not an easy undertaking and he suffered several setbacks at the beginning. Others would have given up but not Dr. Neo. Instead, the problems made him more determined to pursue his goal. He was able to overcome and learn from the obstacles he faced. He even completed a course at the Institute of Leadership and Management to improve his marketing skills. The problems that he experienced in running his business led him to write 3 books on network marketing. He hoped that through his writings, he could guide others to succeed in their businesses.

Busy as Dr. Neo's life is, he still finds time to maintain an ideal work-life balance by engaging with his favourite sports of crossfit and martial arts. He also has hobbies that include shooting on skeet and sporting.

As if all these activities are not enough to fill his day, he also looks after his 16,000 pigs in his full-time piggery farm business, so far the biggest in the Mediterranean. He runs a biogas station as well, thus providing electricity to the community.

Of course, above all his accomplishments, Dr. Neo is foremost a dedicated family man and a loving father to his two lovely daughters who are the jewels of his life.

For more information and to contact Dr. Neo, please visit:

www.DrNeoHealing.com

REFERENCES

1. Halliwell B. How to characterize an antioxidant- an update. Biochem Soc Symp 1995:61:73-101

2. Niki E. Antioxidant defences in eukaryotic cells. In Poli G, Albano E, Dianzani MU, editors: free radicals From Basic science to medicine. Basel, Switzerland: Birkhauser Verlag; 1993. Pp 365-73.

3. Zelko I, Mariani T, folz R. Superoxide dismutase multigene gamily: a comparison of the CuZn-SOD. Free Radical Biological Medicine 2002:33:337-49

4. Wuerges J, Lee JW, Yim YI, Yim HS, Kang SO, Djinovic Carugo K. Crystal structure of Nickel-containing superoxide dismutase reveals another type of active site. Proc natl Acad Sci. 2004:101:8569-74.

5. Chelikani P, Fita I, Loewen PC. Diversity of structures and properties among catalases. Cell Mol. Life Science 2004:61:192-208

6. Matill HA. Antioxidants. Annu Rev Biochem. 1947:16:177-92

7. Caniato R, Filippini R, Piovan A, Puricelli L, Borsarini A, Cappelletti E. Melatonin in plants. Adv. Exp Med Biol. 2003:527:593-7

8. Tan DX, Manchester LC, Reiter RJ, Qi WB, Karbownik M, Calvo JR. Significance of melatonin in antioxidative defense system: Reactions and products. Biol Signals Recept. 2000:9:137-59.

9. Traber MG, Atkinson J. Vitamin E, antioxidant and nothing more. Free Radical Biological Medicine 2007:43:4-15

10. Devasagayam TP, Tilak JC, Boloor KK, Sane KS, Ghaskadbi SS, Lele RD. Free radicals and antioxidants in Human Health: Current status and future prospects. J Assoc Physicians India, 2004:52:794-803